This Diabetes Log Book Belongs to

_____

© and Published by Bold Visions LLC

Introduction

The goal of this log book is to help you track all the health factors involved in managing your diabetes.

Each day has a two-page spread. On the first page you can track:
- Blood sugar
- Insulin dose and other medications
- Blood pressure
- Sleep

The second page is for tracking your food intake and exercise.

Blood Pressure Tracking

Here are the American Heart Association instructions for taking your blood pressure:

- Measure your blood pressure twice a day—morning and late afternoon—at about the same times every day.

- For best results, sit comfortably with both feet on the floor for at least two minutes before taking a measurement.

- To measure your blood pressure, rest your arm on a table so the blood pressure cuff is at about the same height as your heart.

Each day has a place to record your blood pressure. Also, in the back of this book is a table where you can compile the readings into one list, if you want to. Doing so is an easy way to see trends and also an easy log to show your doctor.

SIMPLE WEIGHT TRACKER

DATE	TIME	WEIGHT	NOTES / COMMENTS

Notes

Date _____

	Breakfast		Lunch		Dinner		Bedtime
	Pre	Post	Pre	Post	Pre	Post	
Blood Sugar							
Time							
Insulin Dose							
Medications							

	AM	PM
Blood Pressure		

Sleep Tracking

I went to bed last night at
I got out of bed this morning at
Last night I fell asleep:
    ☐ Easily ☐ After some time ☐ With difficulty
I woke up during the night:
    # of times _____ # of minutes_____
I slept a total of _____ hours
My sleep was disturbed by:

When I woke up for the day, I felt:
    ☐ Refreshed ☐ Somewhat refreshed ☐ Fatigued

Notes
_____
_____
_____

Food Tracking

Breakfast	Servings	Calories	Carbs
Snack			
Lunch			
Snack			
Dinner			
Snack			
TOTAL			

Exercise Tracking

Date _____

	Breakfast		Lunch		Dinner		Bedtime
	Pre	Post	Pre	Post	Pre	Post	
Blood Sugar							
Time							
Insulin Dose							
Medications							

	AM	PM
Blood Pressure		

Sleep Tracking

I went to bed last night at
I got out of bed this morning at
Last night I fell asleep:
☐ Easily ☐ After some time ☐ With difficulty
I woke up during the night:
# of times _____   # of minutes _____
I slept a total of _____ hours
My sleep was disturbed by:

When I woke up for the day, I felt:
☐ Refreshed ☐ Somewhat refreshed ☐ Fatigued

Notes
_____
_____
_____

Food Tracking

Breakfast	Servings	Calories	Carbs
Snack			
Lunch			
Snack			
Dinner			
Snack			
	TOTAL		

Exercise Tracking

Date _____

| | Breakfast || Lunch || Dinner || Bedtime |
	Pre	Post	Pre	Post	Pre	Post	
Blood Sugar							
Time							
Insulin Dose							
Medications							

	AM	PM
Blood Pressure		

Sleep Tracking

I went to bed last night at
I got out of bed this morning at
Last night I fell asleep:
☐ Easily ☐ After some time ☐ With difficulty
I woke up during the night:
# of times _____ # of minutes_____
I slept a total of _____ hours
My sleep was disturbed by:

When I woke up for the day, I felt:
☐ Refreshed ☐ Somewhat refreshed ☐ Fatigued

Notes

_____
_____
_____

Food Tracking

Breakfast	Servings	Calories	Carbs
Snack			
Lunch			
Snack			
Dinner			
Snack			
TOTAL			

Exercise Tracking

Date _____

	Breakfast		Lunch		Dinner		Bedtime
	Pre	Post	Pre	Post	Pre	Post	
Blood Sugar							
Time							
Insulin Dose							
Medications							

	AM	PM
Blood Pressure		

Sleep Tracking

I went to bed last night at
I got out of bed this morning at
Last night I fell asleep:
    ☐ Easily ☐ After some time ☐ With difficulty
I woke up during the night:
    # of times _____ # of minutes_____
I slept a total of _____ hours
My sleep was disturbed by:

When I woke up for the day, I felt:
    ☐ Refreshed ☐ Somewhat refreshed ☐ Fatigued

Notes
_____
_____

Food Tracking

Breakfast	Servings	Calories	Carbs
Snack			
Lunch			
Snack			
Dinner			
Snack			
	TOTAL		

Exercise Tracking

Date _____

| | Breakfast || Lunch || Dinner || Bedtime |
	Pre	Post	Pre	Post	Pre	Post	
Blood Sugar							
Time							
Insulin Dose							
Medications							

	AM	PM
Blood Pressure		

Sleep Tracking

I went to bed last night at
I got out of bed this morning at
Last night I fell asleep:
    ☐ Easily ☐ After some time ☐ With difficulty
I woke up during the night:
    # of times _____ # of minutes_____
I slept a total of _____ hours
My sleep was disturbed by:

When I woke up for the day, I felt:
    ☐ Refreshed ☐ Somewhat refreshed ☐ Fatigued

Notes

_____
_____
_____

Food Tracking

Breakfast	Servings	Calories	Carbs
Snack			
Lunch			
Snack			
Dinner			
Snack			
	TOTAL		

Exercise Tracking

Date _____

| | Breakfast || Lunch || Dinner || Bedtime |
	Pre	Post	Pre	Post	Pre	Post	
Blood Sugar							
Time							
Insulin Dose							
Medications							

	AM	PM
Blood Pressure		

Sleep Tracking

I went to bed last night at
I got out of bed this morning at
Last night I fell asleep:
    ☐ Easily   ☐ After some time   ☐ With difficulty
I woke up during the night:
    # of times _____   # of minutes_____
I slept a total of _____ hours
My sleep was disturbed by:

When I woke up for the day, I felt:
    ☐ Refreshed   ☐ Somewhat refreshed   ☐ Fatigued

Notes

_____
_____

Food Tracking

Breakfast	Servings	Calories	Carbs
Snack			
Lunch			
Snack			
Dinner			
Snack			
TOTAL			

Exercise Tracking

_____

_____

_____

_____

_____

Date _____

| | Breakfast || Lunch || Dinner || Bedtime |
	Pre	Post	Pre	Post	Pre	Post	
Blood Sugar							
Time							
Insulin Dose							
Medications							

	AM	PM
Blood Pressure		

Sleep Tracking

I went to bed last night at
I got out of bed this morning at
Last night I fell asleep:
　　☐ Easily　☐ After some time　☐ With difficulty
I woke up during the night:
　　# of times _____　# of minutes _____
I slept a total of _____ hours
My sleep was disturbed by:

When I woke up for the day, I felt:
　　☐ Refreshed　☐ Somewhat refreshed　☐ Fatigued

Notes

_____
_____
_____

Food Tracking

Breakfast	Servings	Calories	Carbs
Snack			
Lunch			
Snack			
Dinner			
Snack			
	TOTAL		

Exercise Tracking

Date _____

	Breakfast		Lunch		Dinner		Bedtime
	Pre	Post	Pre	Post	Pre	Post	
Blood Sugar							
Time							
Insulin Dose							
Medications							

	AM	PM
Blood Pressure		

Sleep Tracking

I went to bed last night at
I got out of bed this morning at
Last night I fell asleep:
    ☐ Easily ☐ After some time ☐ With difficulty
I woke up during the night:
    # of times _____ # of minutes_____
I slept a total of _____ hours
My sleep was disturbed by:

When I woke up for the day, I felt:
    ☐ Refreshed ☐ Somewhat refreshed ☐ Fatigued

Notes
_____
_____
_____

Food Tracking

Breakfast	Servings	Calories	Carbs
Snack			
Lunch			
Snack			
Dinner			
Snack			
	TOTAL		

Exercise Tracking

Date _____

| | Breakfast || Lunch || Dinner || Bedtime |
	Pre	Post	Pre	Post	Pre	Post	
Blood Sugar							
Time							
Insulin Dose							
Medications							

	AM	PM
Blood Pressure		

Sleep Tracking

I went to bed last night at
I got out of bed this morning at
Last night I fell asleep:
    ☐ Easily ☐ After some time ☐ With difficulty
I woke up during the night:
    # of times _____ # of minutes_____
I slept a total of _____ hours
My sleep was disturbed by:

When I woke up for the day, I felt:
    ☐ Refreshed ☐ Somewhat refreshed ☐ Fatigued

Notes

_____
_____
_____

Food Tracking

Breakfast	Servings	Calories	Carbs
Snack			
Lunch			
Snack			
Dinner			
Snack			
	TOTAL		

Exercise Tracking

Date _____

	Breakfast		Lunch		Dinner		Bedtime
	Pre	Post	Pre	Post	Pre	Post	
Blood Sugar							
Time							
Insulin Dose							
Medications							

	AM	PM
Blood Pressure		

Sleep Tracking

I went to bed last night at
I got out of bed this morning at
Last night I fell asleep:
 ☐ Easily   ☐ After some time   ☐ With difficulty
I woke up during the night:
 # of times _____   # of minutes_____
I slept a total of _____ hours
My sleep was disturbed by:

When I woke up for the day, I felt:
 ☐ Refreshed   ☐ Somewhat refreshed   ☐ Fatigued

Notes
_____
_____
_____

Food Tracking

Breakfast	Servings	Calories	Carbs
Snack			
Lunch			
Snack			
Dinner			
Snack			
	TOTAL		

Exercise Tracking

_____
_____
_____
_____
_____
_____

Date _____

	Breakfast		Lunch		Dinner		Bedtime
	Pre	Post	Pre	Post	Pre	Post	
Blood Sugar							
Time							
Insulin Dose							
Medications							

	AM	PM
Blood Pressure		

Sleep Tracking

I went to bed last night at
I got out of bed this morning at
Last night I fell asleep:
    ☐ Easily ☐ After some time ☐ With difficulty
I woke up during the night:
    # of times _____ # of minutes _____
I slept a total of _____ hours
My sleep was disturbed by:

When I woke up for the day, I felt:
    ☐ Refreshed ☐ Somewhat refreshed ☐ Fatigued

Notes

_____
_____
_____

Food Tracking

Breakfast	Servings	Calories	Carbs
Snack			
Lunch			
Snack			
Dinner			
Snack			
	TOTAL		

Exercise Tracking

Date _____

	Breakfast		Lunch		Dinner		Bedtime
	Pre	Post	Pre	Post	Pre	Post	
Blood Sugar							
Time							
Insulin Dose							
Medications							

	AM	PM
Blood Pressure		

Sleep Tracking

I went to bed last night at
I got out of bed this morning at
Last night I fell asleep:
　　　☐ Easily　☐ After some time　☐ With difficulty
I woke up during the night:
　　　# of times _____　# of minutes _____
I slept a total of _____ hours
My sleep was disturbed by:

When I woke up for the day, I felt:
　　　☐ Refreshed　☐ Somewhat refreshed　☐ Fatigued

Notes
_____
_____
_____

Food Tracking

Breakfast	Servings	Calories	Carbs
Snack			
Lunch			
Snack			
Dinner			
Snack			
	TOTAL		

Exercise Tracking

Date _____

	Breakfast		Lunch		Dinner		Bedtime
	Pre	Post	Pre	Post	Pre	Post	
Blood Sugar							
Time							
Insulin Dose							
Medications							

	AM	PM
Blood Pressure		

Sleep Tracking

I went to bed last night at
I got out of bed this morning at
Last night I fell asleep:
    ☐ Easily ☐ After some time ☐ With difficulty
I woke up during the night:
    # of times _____ # of minutes_____
I slept a total of _____ hours
My sleep was disturbed by:

When I woke up for the day, I felt:
    ☐ Refreshed ☐ Somewhat refreshed ☐ Fatigued

Notes

_____
_____
_____

Food Tracking

Breakfast	Servings	Calories	Carbs
Snack			
Lunch			
Snack			
Dinner			
Snack			
TOTAL			

Exercise Tracking

Date _____

	Breakfast		Lunch		Dinner		Bedtime
	Pre	Post	Pre	Post	Pre	Post	
Blood Sugar							
Time							
Insulin Dose							
Medications							

	AM	PM
Blood Pressure		

Sleep Tracking

I went to bed last night at
I got out of bed this morning at
Last night I fell asleep:
    ☐ Easily ☐ After some time ☐ With difficulty
I woke up during the night:
    # of times _____ # of minutes_____
I slept a total of _____ hours
My sleep was disturbed by:

When I woke up for the day, I felt:
    ☐ Refreshed ☐ Somewhat refreshed ☐ Fatigued

Notes
_____
_____
_____

Food Tracking

Breakfast	Servings	Calories	Carbs
Snack			
Lunch			
Snack			
Dinner			
Snack			
TOTAL			

Exercise Tracking

Date _____

| | Breakfast || Lunch || Dinner || Bedtime |
	Pre	Post	Pre	Post	Pre	Post	
Blood Sugar							
Time							
Insulin Dose							
Medications							

	AM	PM
Blood Pressure		

Sleep Tracking

I went to bed last night at
I got out of bed this morning at
Last night I fell asleep:
    ☐ Easily ☐ After some time ☐ With difficulty
I woke up during the night:
    # of times _____ # of minutes_____
I slept a total of _____ hours
My sleep was disturbed by:

When I woke up for the day, I felt:
    ☐ Refreshed ☐ Somewhat refreshed ☐ Fatigued

Notes

_____
_____
_____

Food Tracking

Breakfast	Servings	Calories	Carbs
Snack			
Lunch			
Snack			
Dinner			
Snack			
	TOTAL		

Exercise Tracking

Date _____

| | Breakfast || Lunch || Dinner || Bedtime |
	Pre	Post	Pre	Post	Pre	Post	
Blood Sugar							
Time							
Insulin Dose							
Medications							

	AM	PM
Blood Pressure		

Sleep Tracking

I went to bed last night at
I got out of bed this morning at
Last night I fell asleep:
  ☐ Easily ☐ After some time ☐ With difficulty
I woke up during the night:
  # of times _____ # of minutes_____
I slept a total of _____ hours
My sleep was disturbed by:

When I woke up for the day, I felt:
  ☐ Refreshed ☐ Somewhat refreshed ☐ Fatigued

Notes

_____
_____
_____

Food Tracking

Breakfast	Servings	Calories	Carbs
Snack			
Lunch			
Snack			
Dinner			
Snack			
TOTAL			

Exercise Tracking

Date _____

	Breakfast		Lunch		Dinner		Bedtime
	Pre	Post	Pre	Post	Pre	Post	
Blood Sugar							
Time							
Insulin Dose							
Medications							

	AM	PM
Blood Pressure		

Sleep Tracking

I went to bed last night at
I got out of bed this morning at
Last night I fell asleep:
    ☐ Easily   ☐ After some time   ☐ With difficulty
I woke up during the night:
    # of times _____   # of minutes_____
I slept a total of _____ hours
My sleep was disturbed by:

When I woke up for the day, I felt:
    ☐ Refreshed   ☐ Somewhat refreshed   ☐ Fatigued

Notes
_____
_____

Food Tracking

Breakfast	Servings	Calories	Carbs
Snack			
Lunch			
Snack			
Dinner			
Snack			
	TOTAL		

Exercise Tracking

Date _____

	Breakfast		Lunch		Dinner		Bedtime
	Pre	Post	Pre	Post	Pre	Post	
Blood Sugar							
Time							
Insulin Dose							
Medications							

	AM	PM
Blood Pressure		

Sleep Tracking

I went to bed last night at
I got out of bed this morning at
Last night I fell asleep:
    ☐ Easily ☐ After some time ☐ With difficulty
I woke up during the night:
    # of times _____ # of minutes_____
I slept a total of _____ hours
My sleep was disturbed by:

When I woke up for the day, I felt:
    ☐ Refreshed ☐ Somewhat refreshed ☐ Fatigued

Notes
_____
_____
_____

Food Tracking

Breakfast	Servings	Calories	Carbs
Snack			
Lunch			
Snack			
Dinner			
Snack			
	TOTAL		

Exercise Tracking

Date _____

| | Breakfast || Lunch || Dinner || Bedtime |
	Pre	Post	Pre	Post	Pre	Post	
Blood Sugar							
Time							
Insulin Dose							
Medications							

	AM	PM
Blood Pressure		

Sleep Tracking

I went to bed last night at
I got out of bed this morning at
Last night I fell asleep:
    ☐ Easily   ☐ After some time   ☐ With difficulty
I woke up during the night:
    # of times _____   # of minutes_____
I slept a total of _____ hours
My sleep was disturbed by:

When I woke up for the day, I felt:
    ☐ Refreshed   ☐ Somewhat refreshed   ☐ Fatigued

Notes
_____
_____

Food Tracking

Breakfast	Servings	Calories	Carbs
Snack			
Lunch			
Snack			
Dinner			
Snack			
	TOTAL		

Exercise Tracking

Date _____

	Breakfast		Lunch		Dinner		Bedtime
	Pre	Post	Pre	Post	Pre	Post	
Blood Sugar							
Time							
Insulin Dose							
Medications							

	AM	PM
Blood Pressure		

Sleep Tracking

I went to bed last night at
I got out of bed this morning at
Last night I fell asleep:
    ☐ Easily ☐ After some time ☐ With difficulty
I woke up during the night:
    # of times _____ # of minutes_____
I slept a total of _____ hours
My sleep was disturbed by:

When I woke up for the day, I felt:
    ☐ Refreshed ☐ Somewhat refreshed ☐ Fatigued

Notes
_____
_____
_____

Food Tracking

Breakfast	Servings	Calories	Carbs
Snack			
Lunch			
Snack			
Dinner			
Snack			
	TOTAL		

Exercise Tracking

Date _____

	Breakfast		Lunch		Dinner		Bedtime
	Pre	Post	Pre	Post	Pre	Post	
Blood Sugar							
Time							
Insulin Dose							
Medications							

	AM	PM
Blood Pressure		

Sleep Tracking

I went to bed last night at
I got out of bed this morning at
Last night I fell asleep:
    ☐ Easily ☐ After some time ☐ With difficulty
I woke up during the night:
    # of times _____ # of minutes_____
I slept a total of _____ hours
My sleep was disturbed by:

When I woke up for the day, I felt:
    ☐ Refreshed ☐ Somewhat refreshed ☐ Fatigued

Notes

_____
_____
_____

Food Tracking

Breakfast	Servings	Calories	Carbs
Snack			
Lunch			
Snack			
Dinner			
Snack			
	TOTAL		

Exercise Tracking

Date _____

	Breakfast		Lunch		Dinner		Bedtime
	Pre	Post	Pre	Post	Pre	Post	
Blood Sugar							
Time							
Insulin Dose							
Medications							

	AM	PM
Blood Pressure		

Sleep Tracking

I went to bed last night at
I got out of bed this morning at
Last night I fell asleep:
 ☐ Easily ☐ After some time ☐ With difficulty
I woke up during the night:
 # of times _____ # of minutes _____
I slept a total of _____ hours
My sleep was disturbed by:

When I woke up for the day, I felt:
 ☐ Refreshed ☐ Somewhat refreshed ☐ Fatigued

Notes
_____
_____

Food Tracking

Breakfast	Servings	Calories	Carbs
Snack			
Lunch			
Snack			
Dinner			
Snack			
	TOTAL		

Exercise Tracking

Date _____

| | Breakfast || Lunch || Dinner || Bedtime |
	Pre	Post	Pre	Post	Pre	Post	
Blood Sugar							
Time							
Insulin Dose							
Medications							

	AM	PM
Blood Pressure		

Sleep Tracking

I went to bed last night at
I got out of bed this morning at
Last night I fell asleep:
    ☐ Easily ☐ After some time ☐ With difficulty
I woke up during the night:
    # of times _____   # of minutes_____
I slept a total of _____ hours
My sleep was disturbed by:

When I woke up for the day, I felt:
    ☐ Refreshed ☐ Somewhat refreshed ☐ Fatigued

Notes

_____
_____
_____

Food Tracking

Breakfast	Servings	Calories	Carbs
Snack			
Lunch			
Snack			
Dinner			
Snack			
	TOTAL		

Exercise Tracking

Date _____

| | Breakfast || Lunch || Dinner || Bedtime |
	Pre	Post	Pre	Post	Pre	Post	
Blood Sugar							
Time							
Insulin Dose							
Medications							

	AM	PM
Blood Pressure		

Sleep Tracking

I went to bed last night at
I got out of bed this morning at
Last night I fell asleep:
    ☐ Easily ☐ After some time ☐ With difficulty
I woke up during the night:
    # of times _____ # of minutes_____
I slept a total of _____ hours
My sleep was disturbed by:

When I woke up for the day, I felt:
    ☐ Refreshed ☐ Somewhat refreshed ☐ Fatigued

Notes
_____
_____

Food Tracking

Breakfast	Servings	Calories	Carbs
Snack			
Lunch			
Snack			
Dinner			
Snack			
TOTAL			

Exercise Tracking

Date _____

| | Breakfast || Lunch || Dinner || Bedtime |
	Pre	Post	Pre	Post	Pre	Post	
Blood Sugar							
Time							
Insulin Dose							
Medications							

	AM	PM
Blood Pressure		

Sleep Tracking

I went to bed last night at
I got out of bed this morning at
Last night I fell asleep:
    ☐ Easily ☐ After some time ☐ With difficulty
I woke up during the night:
    # of times _____ # of minutes_____
I slept a total of _____ hours
My sleep was disturbed by:

When I woke up for the day, I felt:
    ☐ Refreshed ☐ Somewhat refreshed ☐ Fatigued

Notes

_____
_____
_____

Food Tracking

Breakfast	Servings	Calories	Carbs
Snack			
Lunch			
Snack			
Dinner			
Snack			
TOTAL			

Exercise Tracking

Date _____

| | Breakfast || Lunch || Dinner || Bedtime |
	Pre	Post	Pre	Post	Pre	Post	
Blood Sugar							
Time							
Insulin Dose							
Medications							

	AM	PM
Blood Pressure		

Sleep Tracking

I went to bed last night at
I got out of bed this morning at
Last night I fell asleep:
　　　☐ Easily　☐ After some time　☐ With difficulty
I woke up during the night:
　　　# of times _____　# of minutes _____
I slept a total of _____ hours
My sleep was disturbed by:

When I woke up for the day, I felt:
　　　☐ Refreshed　☐ Somewhat refreshed　☐ Fatigued

Notes
_____
_____
_____

Food Tracking

Breakfast	Servings	Calories	Carbs
Snack			
Lunch			
Snack			
Dinner			
Snack			
	TOTAL		

Exercise Tracking

Date _____

| | Breakfast || Lunch || Dinner || Bedtime |
	Pre	Post	Pre	Post	Pre	Post	
Blood Sugar							
Time							
Insulin Dose							
Medications							

	AM	PM
Blood Pressure		

Sleep Tracking

I went to bed last night at
I got out of bed this morning at
Last night I fell asleep:
    ☐ Easily ☐ After some time ☐ With difficulty
I woke up during the night:
    # of times _____   # of minutes_____
I slept a total of _____ hours
My sleep was disturbed by:

When I woke up for the day, I felt:
    ☐ Refreshed ☐ Somewhat refreshed ☐ Fatigued

Notes
_____
_____
_____

Food Tracking

Breakfast	Servings	Calories	Carbs
Snack			
Lunch			
Snack			
Dinner			
Snack			
	TOTAL		

Exercise Tracking

Date _____

| | Breakfast || Lunch || Dinner || Bedtime |
	Pre	Post	Pre	Post	Pre	Post	
Blood Sugar							
Time							
Insulin Dose							
Medications							

	AM	PM
Blood Pressure		

Sleep Tracking

I went to bed last night at
I got out of bed this morning at
Last night I fell asleep:
    ☐ Easily ☐ After some time ☐ With difficulty
I woke up during the night:
    # of times _____ # of minutes_____
I slept a total of _____ hours
My sleep was disturbed by:

When I woke up for the day, I felt:
    ☐ Refreshed ☐ Somewhat refreshed ☐ Fatigued

Notes
_____
_____
_____

Food Tracking

Breakfast	Servings	Calories	Carbs
Snack			
Lunch			
Snack			
Dinner			
Snack			
	TOTAL		

Exercise Tracking

Date _____

| | Breakfast || Lunch || Dinner || Bedtime |
	Pre	Post	Pre	Post	Pre	Post	
Blood Sugar							
Time							
Insulin Dose							
Medications							

	AM	PM
Blood Pressure		

Sleep Tracking

I went to bed last night at
I got out of bed this morning at
Last night I fell asleep:
    ☐ Easily ☐ After some time ☐ With difficulty
I woke up during the night:
    # of times _____ # of minutes_____
I slept a total of _____ hours
My sleep was disturbed by:

When I woke up for the day, I felt:
    ☐ Refreshed ☐ Somewhat refreshed ☐ Fatigued

Notes
_____
_____
_____

Food Tracking

Breakfast	Servings	Calories	Carbs
Snack			
Lunch			
Snack			
Dinner			
Snack			
	TOTAL		

Exercise Tracking

Date _____

| | Breakfast || Lunch || Dinner || Bedtime |
	Pre	Post	Pre	Post	Pre	Post	
Blood Sugar							
Time							
Insulin Dose							
Medications							

	AM	PM
Blood Pressure		

Sleep Tracking

I went to bed last night at
I got out of bed this morning at
Last night I fell asleep:
    ☐ Easily ☐ After some time ☐ With difficulty
I woke up during the night:
    # of times _____ # of minutes_____
I slept a total of _____ hours
My sleep was disturbed by:

When I woke up for the day, I felt:
    ☐ Refreshed ☐ Somewhat refreshed ☐ Fatigued

Notes
_____
_____

Food Tracking

Breakfast	Servings	Calories	Carbs
Snack			
Lunch			
Snack			
Dinner			
Snack			
TOTAL			

Exercise Tracking

Date _____

	Breakfast		Lunch		Dinner		Bedtime
	Pre	Post	Pre	Post	Pre	Post	
Blood Sugar							
Time							
Insulin Dose							
Medications							

	AM	PM
Blood Pressure		

Sleep Tracking

I went to bed last night at
I got out of bed this morning at
Last night I fell asleep:
☐ Easily ☐ After some time ☐ With difficulty
I woke up during the night:
# of times _____   # of minutes_____
I slept a total of _____ hours
My sleep was disturbed by:

When I woke up for the day, I felt:
☐ Refreshed ☐ Somewhat refreshed ☐ Fatigued

Notes
_____
_____
_____

Food Tracking

Breakfast	Servings	Calories	Carbs
Snack			
Lunch			
Snack			
Dinner			
Snack			
	TOTAL		

Exercise Tracking

Date _____

| | Breakfast || Lunch || Dinner || Bedtime |
	Pre	Post	Pre	Post	Pre	Post	
Blood Sugar							
Time							
Insulin Dose							
Medications							

	AM	PM
Blood Pressure		

Sleep Tracking

I went to bed last night at
I got out of bed this morning at
Last night I fell asleep:
  ☐ Easily ☐ After some time ☐ With difficulty
I woke up during the night:
  # of times _____   # of minutes_____
I slept a total of _____ hours
My sleep was disturbed by:

When I woke up for the day, I felt:
  ☐ Refreshed ☐ Somewhat refreshed ☐ Fatigued

Notes
_____
_____
_____

Food Tracking

Breakfast	Servings	Calories	Carbs
Snack			
Lunch			
Snack			
Dinner			
Snack			
TOTAL			

Exercise Tracking

Date _____

	Breakfast		Lunch		Dinner		Bedtime
	Pre	Post	Pre	Post	Pre	Post	
Blood Sugar							
Time							
Insulin Dose							
Medications							

	AM	PM
Blood Pressure		

Sleep Tracking

I went to bed last night at
I got out of bed this morning at
Last night I fell asleep:
    ☐ Easily ☐ After some time ☐ With difficulty
I woke up during the night:
    # of times _____ # of minutes_____
I slept a total of _____ hours
My sleep was disturbed by:

When I woke up for the day, I felt:
    ☐ Refreshed ☐ Somewhat refreshed ☐ Fatigued

Notes
_____
_____
_____

Food Tracking

Breakfast	Servings	Calories	Carbs
Snack			
Lunch			
Snack			
Dinner			
Snack			
	TOTAL		

Exercise Tracking

Date _____

	Breakfast		Lunch		Dinner		Bedtime
	Pre	Post	Pre	Post	Pre	Post	
Blood Sugar							
Time							
Insulin Dose							
Medications							

	AM	PM
Blood Pressure		

Sleep Tracking

I went to bed last night at
I got out of bed this morning at
Last night I fell asleep:
☐ Easily ☐ After some time ☐ With difficulty
I woke up during the night:
# of times _____ # of minutes_____
I slept a total of _____ hours
My sleep was disturbed by:

When I woke up for the day, I felt:
☐ Refreshed ☐ Somewhat refreshed ☐ Fatigued

Notes
_____
_____
_____

Food Tracking

Breakfast	Servings	Calories	Carbs
Snack			
Lunch			
Snack			
Dinner			
Snack			
TOTAL			

Exercise Tracking

Date _____

| | Breakfast || Lunch || Dinner || Bedtime |
	Pre	Post	Pre	Post	Pre	Post	
Blood Sugar							
Time							
Insulin Dose							
Medications							

	AM	PM
Blood Pressure		

Sleep Tracking

I went to bed last night at
I got out of bed this morning at
Last night I fell asleep:
    ☐ Easily ☐ After some time ☐ With difficulty
I woke up during the night:
    # of times _____ # of minutes_____
I slept a total of _____ hours
My sleep was disturbed by:

When I woke up for the day, I felt:
    ☐ Refreshed ☐ Somewhat refreshed ☐ Fatigued

Notes
_____
_____
_____

Food Tracking

Breakfast	Servings	Calories	Carbs
Snack			
Lunch			
Snack			
Dinner			
Snack			
	TOTAL		

Exercise Tracking

Date _____

	Breakfast		Lunch		Dinner		Bedtime
	Pre	Post	Pre	Post	Pre	Post	
Blood Sugar							
Time							
Insulin Dose							
Medications							

	AM	PM
Blood Pressure		

Sleep Tracking

I went to bed last night at
I got out of bed this morning at
Last night I fell asleep:
　　☐ Easily ☐ After some time ☐ With difficulty
I woke up during the night:
　　# of times _____   # of minutes_____
I slept a total of _____ hours
My sleep was disturbed by:

When I woke up for the day, I felt:
　　☐ Refreshed ☐ Somewhat refreshed ☐ Fatigued

Notes
_____
_____
_____

Food Tracking

Breakfast	Servings	Calories	Carbs
Snack			
Lunch			
Snack			
Dinner			
Snack			
	TOTAL		

Exercise Tracking

Date _____

| | Breakfast || Lunch || Dinner || Bedtime |
	Pre	Post	Pre	Post	Pre	Post	
Blood Sugar							
Time							
Insulin Dose							
Medications							

	AM	PM
Blood Pressure		

Sleep Tracking

I went to bed last night at
I got out of bed this morning at
Last night I fell asleep:
 ☐ Easily ☐ After some time ☐ With difficulty
I woke up during the night:
 # of times _____ # of minutes_____
I slept a total of _____ hours
My sleep was disturbed by:

When I woke up for the day, I felt:
 ☐ Refreshed ☐ Somewhat refreshed ☐ Fatigued

Notes
_____
_____
_____

Food Tracking

Breakfast	Servings	Calories	Carbs
Snack			
Lunch			
Snack			
Dinner			
Snack			
TOTAL			

Exercise Tracking

Date _____

| | Breakfast || Lunch || Dinner || Bedtime |
	Pre	Post	Pre	Post	Pre	Post	
Blood Sugar							
Time							
Insulin Dose							
Medications							

	AM	PM
Blood Pressure		

Sleep Tracking

I went to bed last night at
I got out of bed this morning at
Last night I fell asleep:
 ☐ Easily ☐ After some time ☐ With difficulty
I woke up during the night:
 # of times _____ # of minutes _____
I slept a total of _____ hours
My sleep was disturbed by:

When I woke up for the day, I felt:
 ☐ Refreshed ☐ Somewhat refreshed ☐ Fatigued

Notes

_____
_____
_____

Food Tracking

Breakfast	Servings	Calories	Carbs
Snack			
Lunch			
Snack			
Dinner			
Snack			
	TOTAL		

Exercise Tracking

_____
_____
_____
_____
_____

Date _____

	Breakfast		Lunch		Dinner		Bedtime
	Pre	Post	Pre	Post	Pre	Post	
Blood Sugar							
Time							
Insulin Dose							
Medications							

	AM	PM
Blood Pressure		

Sleep Tracking

I went to bed last night at
I got out of bed this morning at
Last night I fell asleep:
☐ Easily ☐ After some time ☐ With difficulty
I woke up during the night:
\# of times _____   # of minutes_____
I slept a total of _____ hours
My sleep was disturbed by:

When I woke up for the day, I felt:
☐ Refreshed ☐ Somewhat refreshed ☐ Fatigued

Notes
_____
_____
_____

Food Tracking

Breakfast	Servings	Calories	Carbs
Snack			
Lunch			
Snack			
Dinner			
Snack			
	TOTAL		

Exercise Tracking

_____
_____
_____
_____
_____

Date _____

	Breakfast		Lunch		Dinner		Bedtime
	Pre	Post	Pre	Post	Pre	Post	
Blood Sugar							
Time							
Insulin Dose							
Medications							

	AM	PM
Blood Pressure		

Sleep Tracking

I went to bed last night at
I got out of bed this morning at
Last night I fell asleep:
☐ Easily ☐ After some time ☐ With difficulty
I woke up during the night:
\# of times _____ # of minutes_____
I slept a total of _____ hours
My sleep was disturbed by:

When I woke up for the day, I felt:
☐ Refreshed ☐ Somewhat refreshed ☐ Fatigued

Notes
_____
_____

Food Tracking

Breakfast	Servings	Calories	Carbs
Snack			
Lunch			
Snack			
Dinner			
Snack			
	TOTAL		

Exercise Tracking

Date _____

	Breakfast		Lunch		Dinner		Bedtime
	Pre	Post	Pre	Post	Pre	Post	
Blood Sugar							
Time							
Insulin Dose							
Medications							

	AM	PM
Blood Pressure		

Sleep Tracking

I went to bed last night at
I got out of bed this morning at
Last night I fell asleep:
　　　☐ Easily　☐ After some time　☐ With difficulty
I woke up during the night:
　　　# of times _____　# of minutes_____
I slept a total of _____ hours
My sleep was disturbed by:

When I woke up for the day, I felt:
　　　☐ Refreshed　☐ Somewhat refreshed　☐ Fatigued

Notes
_____
_____
_____

Food Tracking

Breakfast	Servings	Calories	Carbs
Snack			
Lunch			
Snack			
Dinner			
Snack			
	TOTAL		

Exercise Tracking

Date _____

| | Breakfast || Lunch || Dinner || Bedtime |
	Pre	Post	Pre	Post	Pre	Post	
Blood Sugar							
Time							
Insulin Dose							
Medications							

	AM	PM
Blood Pressure		

Sleep Tracking

I went to bed last night at
I got out of bed this morning at
Last night I fell asleep:
☐ Easily ☐ After some time ☐ With difficulty
I woke up during the night:
# of times _____ # of minutes _____
I slept a total of _____ hours
My sleep was disturbed by:

When I woke up for the day, I felt:
☐ Refreshed ☐ Somewhat refreshed ☐ Fatigued

Notes
_____
_____
_____

Food Tracking

Breakfast	Servings	Calories	Carbs
Snack			
Lunch			
Snack			
Dinner			
Snack			
	TOTAL		

Exercise Tracking

Date _____

	Breakfast		Lunch		Dinner		Bedtime
	Pre	Post	Pre	Post	Pre	Post	
Blood Sugar							
Time							
Insulin Dose							
Medications							

	AM	PM
Blood Pressure		

Sleep Tracking

I went to bed last night at
I got out of bed this morning at
Last night I fell asleep:
    ☐ Easily ☐ After some time ☐ With difficulty
I woke up during the night:
    # of times _____ # of minutes _____
I slept a total of _____ hours
My sleep was disturbed by:

When I woke up for the day, I felt:
    ☐ Refreshed ☐ Somewhat refreshed ☐ Fatigued

Notes
_____
_____
_____

Food Tracking

Breakfast	Servings	Calories	Carbs
Snack			
Lunch			
Snack			
Dinner			
Snack			
	TOTAL		

Exercise Tracking

Date _____

	Breakfast		Lunch		Dinner		Bedtime
	Pre	Post	Pre	Post	Pre	Post	
Blood Sugar							
Time							
Insulin Dose							
Medications							

	AM	PM
Blood Pressure		

Sleep Tracking

I went to bed last night at
I got out of bed this morning at
Last night I fell asleep:
    ☐ Easily   ☐ After some time   ☐ With difficulty
I woke up during the night:
    # of times _____   # of minutes _____
I slept a total of _____ hours
My sleep was disturbed by:

When I woke up for the day, I felt:
    ☐ Refreshed   ☐ Somewhat refreshed   ☐ Fatigued

Notes
_____
_____
_____

Food Tracking

Breakfast	Servings	Calories	Carbs
Snack			
Lunch			
Snack			
Dinner			
Snack			
	TOTAL		

Exercise Tracking

Date _____

| | Breakfast || Lunch || Dinner || Bedtime |
	Pre	Post	Pre	Post	Pre	Post	
Blood Sugar							
Time							
Insulin Dose							
Medications							

	AM	PM
Blood Pressure		

Sleep Tracking

I went to bed last night at
I got out of bed this morning at
Last night I fell asleep:
    ☐ Easily ☐ After some time ☐ With difficulty
I woke up during the night:
    # of times _____ # of minutes_____
I slept a total of _____ hours
My sleep was disturbed by:

When I woke up for the day, I felt:
    ☐ Refreshed ☐ Somewhat refreshed ☐ Fatigued

Notes
_____
_____

Food Tracking

Breakfast	Servings	Calories	Carbs
Snack			
Lunch			
Snack			
Dinner			
Snack			
	TOTAL		

Exercise Tracking

Date _____

| | Breakfast || Lunch || Dinner || Bedtime |
	Pre	Post	Pre	Post	Pre	Post	
Blood Sugar							
Time							
Insulin Dose							
Medications							

	AM	PM
Blood Pressure		

Sleep Tracking

I went to bed last night at
I got out of bed this morning at
Last night I fell asleep:
    ☐ Easily ☐ After some time ☐ With difficulty
I woke up during the night:
    # of times _____ # of minutes_____
I slept a total of _____ hours
My sleep was disturbed by:

When I woke up for the day, I felt:
    ☐ Refreshed ☐ Somewhat refreshed ☐ Fatigued

Notes
_____
_____
_____

Food Tracking

Breakfast	Servings	Calories	Carbs
Snack			
Lunch			
Snack			
Dinner			
Snack			
TOTAL			

Exercise Tracking

Date _____

| | Breakfast || Lunch || Dinner || Bedtime |
	Pre	Post	Pre	Post	Pre	Post	
Blood Sugar							
Time							
Insulin Dose							
Medications							

	AM	PM
Blood Pressure		

Sleep Tracking

I went to bed last night at
I got out of bed this morning at
Last night I fell asleep:
    ☐ Easily ☐ After some time ☐ With difficulty
I woke up during the night:
    # of times _____ # of minutes_____
I slept a total of _____ hours
My sleep was disturbed by:

When I woke up for the day, I felt:
    ☐ Refreshed ☐ Somewhat refreshed ☐ Fatigued

Notes
_____
_____
_____

Food Tracking

Breakfast	Servings	Calories	Carbs
Snack			
Lunch			
Snack			
Dinner			
Snack			
	TOTAL		

Exercise Tracking

Date _____

	Breakfast		Lunch		Dinner		Bedtime
	Pre	Post	Pre	Post	Pre	Post	
Blood Sugar							
Time							
Insulin Dose							
Medications							

	AM	PM
Blood Pressure		

Sleep Tracking

I went to bed last night at
I got out of bed this morning at
Last night I fell asleep:
  ☐ Easily ☐ After some time ☐ With difficulty
I woke up during the night:
  # of times _____ # of minutes_____
I slept a total of _____ hours
My sleep was disturbed by:

When I woke up for the day, I felt:
  ☐ Refreshed ☐ Somewhat refreshed ☐ Fatigued

Notes
_____
_____
_____

Food Tracking

Breakfast	Servings	Calories	Carbs
Snack			
Lunch			
Snack			
Dinner			
Snack			
	TOTAL		

Exercise Tracking

Date _____

	Breakfast		Lunch		Dinner		Bedtime
	Pre	Post	Pre	Post	Pre	Post	
Blood Sugar							
Time							
Insulin Dose							
Medications							

	AM	PM
Blood Pressure		

Sleep Tracking

I went to bed last night at
I got out of bed this morning at
Last night I fell asleep:
    ☐ Easily   ☐ After some time   ☐ With difficulty
I woke up during the night:
    # of times _____   # of minutes_____
I slept a total of _____ hours
My sleep was disturbed by:

When I woke up for the day, I felt:
    ☐ Refreshed   ☐ Somewhat refreshed   ☐ Fatigued

Notes
_____
_____
_____

Food Tracking

Breakfast	Servings	Calories	Carbs
Snack			
Lunch			
Snack			
Dinner			
Snack			
	TOTAL		

Exercise Tracking

Date _____

	Breakfast		Lunch		Dinner		Bedtime
	Pre	Post	Pre	Post	Pre	Post	
Blood Sugar							
Time							
Insulin Dose							
Medications							

	AM	PM
Blood Pressure		

Sleep Tracking

I went to bed last night at
I got out of bed this morning at
Last night I fell asleep:
    ☐ Easily ☐ After some time ☐ With difficulty
I woke up during the night:
    # of times _____   # of minutes_____
I slept a total of _____ hours
My sleep was disturbed by:

When I woke up for the day, I felt:
    ☐ Refreshed ☐ Somewhat refreshed ☐ Fatigued

Notes
_____
_____
_____

Food Tracking

Breakfast	Servings	Calories	Carbs
Snack			
Lunch			
Snack			
Dinner			
Snack			
	TOTAL		

Exercise Tracking

Date _____

| | Breakfast || Lunch || Dinner || Bedtime |
	Pre	Post	Pre	Post	Pre	Post	
Blood Sugar							
Time							
Insulin Dose							
Medications							

	AM	PM
Blood Pressure		

Sleep Tracking

I went to bed last night at
I got out of bed this morning at
Last night I fell asleep:
    ☐ Easily   ☐ After some time   ☐ With difficulty
I woke up during the night:
    # of times _____   # of minutes_____
I slept a total of _____ hours
My sleep was disturbed by:

When I woke up for the day, I felt:
    ☐ Refreshed   ☐ Somewhat refreshed   ☐ Fatigued

Notes
_____
_____
_____

Food Tracking

Breakfast	Servings	Calories	Carbs
Snack			
Lunch			
Snack			
Dinner			
Snack			
TOTAL			

Exercise Tracking

Date _____

| | Breakfast || Lunch || Dinner || Bedtime |
	Pre	Post	Pre	Post	Pre	Post	
Blood Sugar							
Time							
Insulin Dose							
Medications							

	AM	PM
Blood Pressure		

Sleep Tracking

I went to bed last night at
I got out of bed this morning at
Last night I fell asleep:
    ☐ Easily ☐ After some time ☐ With difficulty
I woke up during the night:
    # of times _____   # of minutes_____
I slept a total of _____ hours
My sleep was disturbed by:

When I woke up for the day, I felt:
    ☐ Refreshed ☐ Somewhat refreshed ☐ Fatigued

Notes
_____
_____
_____

Food Tracking

	Servings	Calories	Carbs
Breakfast			
Snack			
Lunch			
Snack			
Dinner			
Snack			
TOTAL			

Exercise Tracking

Date _____

| | Breakfast || Lunch || Dinner || Bedtime |
	Pre	Post	Pre	Post	Pre	Post	
Blood Sugar							
Time							
Insulin Dose							
Medications							

	AM	PM
Blood Pressure		

Sleep Tracking

I went to bed last night at
I got out of bed this morning at
Last night I fell asleep:
    ☐ Easily   ☐ After some time   ☐ With difficulty
I woke up during the night:
    # of times _____   # of minutes _____
I slept a total of _____ hours
My sleep was disturbed by:

When I woke up for the day, I felt:
    ☐ Refreshed   ☐ Somewhat refreshed   ☐ Fatigued

Notes
_____
_____
_____

Food Tracking

Breakfast	Servings	Calories	Carbs
Snack			
Lunch			
Snack			
Dinner			
Snack			
	TOTAL		

Exercise Tracking

Date _____

	Breakfast		Lunch		Dinner		Bedtime
	Pre	Post	Pre	Post	Pre	Post	
Blood Sugar							
Time							
Insulin Dose							
Medications							

	AM	PM
Blood Pressure		

Sleep Tracking

I went to bed last night at
I got out of bed this morning at
Last night I fell asleep:
    ☐ Easily   ☐ After some time   ☐ With difficulty
I woke up during the night:
    # of times _____   # of minutes_____
I slept a total of _____ hours
My sleep was disturbed by:

When I woke up for the day, I felt:
    ☐ Refreshed   ☐ Somewhat refreshed   ☐ Fatigued

Notes
_____
_____
_____

Food Tracking

Breakfast	Servings	Calories	Carbs
Snack			
Lunch			
Snack			
Dinner			
Snack			
	TOTAL		

Exercise Tracking

Date _____

	Breakfast		Lunch		Dinner		Bedtime
	Pre	Post	Pre	Post	Pre	Post	
Blood Sugar							
Time							
Insulin Dose							
Medications							

	AM	PM
Blood Pressure		

Sleep Tracking

I went to bed last night at
I got out of bed this morning at
Last night I fell asleep:
    ☐ Easily ☐ After some time ☐ With difficulty
I woke up during the night:
    # of times _____ # of minutes_____
I slept a total of _____ hours
My sleep was disturbed by:

When I woke up for the day, I felt:
    ☐ Refreshed ☐ Somewhat refreshed ☐ Fatigued

Notes

_____
_____
_____

Food Tracking

Breakfast	Servings	Calories	Carbs
Snack			
Lunch			
Snack			
Dinner			
Snack			
TOTAL			

Exercise Tracking

Date _____

	Breakfast		Lunch		Dinner		Bedtime
	Pre	Post	Pre	Post	Pre	Post	
Blood Sugar							
Time							
Insulin Dose							
Medications							

	AM	PM
Blood Pressure		

Sleep Tracking

I went to bed last night at
I got out of bed this morning at
Last night I fell asleep:
    ☐ Easily   ☐ After some time   ☐ With difficulty
I woke up during the night:
    # of times _____   # of minutes_____
I slept a total of _____ hours
My sleep was disturbed by:

When I woke up for the day, I felt:
    ☐ Refreshed   ☐ Somewhat refreshed   ☐ Fatigued

Notes

_____
_____
_____

Food Tracking

Breakfast	Servings	Calories	Carbs
Snack			
Lunch			
Snack			
Dinner			
Snack			
	TOTAL		

Exercise Tracking

Date _____

	Breakfast		Lunch		Dinner		Bedtime
	Pre	Post	Pre	Post	Pre	Post	
Blood Sugar							
Time							
Insulin Dose							
Medications							

	AM	PM
Blood Pressure		

Sleep Tracking

I went to bed last night at
I got out of bed this morning at
Last night I fell asleep:
    ☐ Easily   ☐ After some time   ☐ With difficulty
I woke up during the night:
    # of times _____   # of minutes_____
I slept a total of _____ hours
My sleep was disturbed by:

When I woke up for the day, I felt:
    ☐ Refreshed   ☐ Somewhat refreshed   ☐ Fatigued

Notes
_____
_____
_____

Food Tracking

Breakfast	Servings	Calories	Carbs
Snack			
Lunch			
Snack			
Dinner			
Snack			
	TOTAL		

Exercise Tracking

Date _____

	Breakfast		Lunch		Dinner		Bedtime
	Pre	Post	Pre	Post	Pre	Post	
Blood Sugar							
Time							
Insulin Dose							
Medications							

	AM	PM
Blood Pressure		

Sleep Tracking

I went to bed last night at
I got out of bed this morning at
Last night I fell asleep:
    ☐ Easily   ☐ After some time   ☐ With difficulty
I woke up during the night:
    # of times _____   # of minutes_____
I slept a total of _____ hours
My sleep was disturbed by:

When I woke up for the day, I felt:
    ☐ Refreshed   ☐ Somewhat refreshed   ☐ Fatigued

Notes
_____
_____
_____

Food Tracking

Breakfast	Servings	Calories	Carbs
Snack			
Lunch			
Snack			
Dinner			
Snack			
	TOTAL		

Exercise Tracking

Date _____

	Breakfast		Lunch		Dinner		Bedtime
	Pre	Post	Pre	Post	Pre	Post	
Blood Sugar							
Time							
Insulin Dose							
Medications							

	AM	PM
Blood Pressure		

Sleep Tracking

I went to bed last night at
I got out of bed this morning at
Last night I fell asleep:
    ☐ Easily ☐ After some time ☐ With difficulty
I woke up during the night:
    # of times _____ # of minutes_____
I slept a total of _____ hours
My sleep was disturbed by:

When I woke up for the day, I felt:
    ☐ Refreshed ☐ Somewhat refreshed ☐ Fatigued

Notes

_____
_____
_____

Food Tracking

Breakfast	Servings	Calories	Carbs
Snack			
Lunch			
Snack			
Dinner			
Snack			
	TOTAL		

Exercise Tracking

_____
_____
_____
_____
_____

Date _____

| | Breakfast || Lunch || Dinner || Bedtime |
	Pre	Post	Pre	Post	Pre	Post	
Blood Sugar							
Time							
Insulin Dose							
Medications							

	AM	PM
Blood Pressure		

Sleep Tracking

I went to bed last night at
I got out of bed this morning at
Last night I fell asleep:
    ☐ Easily ☐ After some time ☐ With difficulty
I woke up during the night:
    # of times _____ # of minutes_____
I slept a total of _____ hours
My sleep was disturbed by:

When I woke up for the day, I felt:
    ☐ Refreshed ☐ Somewhat refreshed ☐ Fatigued

Notes
_____
_____
_____

Food Tracking

Breakfast	Servings	Calories	Carbs
Snack			
Lunch			
Snack			
Dinner			
Snack			
	TOTAL		

Exercise Tracking

Date _____

	Breakfast		Lunch		Dinner		Bedtime
	Pre	Post	Pre	Post	Pre	Post	
Blood Sugar							
Time							
Insulin Dose							
Medications							

	AM	PM
Blood Pressure		

Sleep Tracking

I went to bed last night at
I got out of bed this morning at
Last night I fell asleep:
    ☐ Easily ☐ After some time ☐ With difficulty
I woke up during the night:
    # of times _____ # of minutes_____
I slept a total of _____ hours
My sleep was disturbed by:

When I woke up for the day, I felt:
    ☐ Refreshed ☐ Somewhat refreshed ☐ Fatigued

Notes
_____
_____
_____

Food Tracking

Breakfast	Servings	Calories	Carbs
Snack			
Lunch			
Snack			
Dinner			
Snack			
TOTAL			

Exercise Tracking

Date _____

	Breakfast		Lunch		Dinner		Bedtime
	Pre	Post	Pre	Post	Pre	Post	
Blood Sugar							
Time							
Insulin Dose							
Medications							

	AM	PM
Blood Pressure		

Sleep Tracking

I went to bed last night at
I got out of bed this morning at
Last night I fell asleep:
    ☐ Easily ☐ After some time ☐ With difficulty
I woke up during the night:
    # of times _____ # of minutes_____
I slept a total of _____ hours
My sleep was disturbed by:

When I woke up for the day, I felt:
    ☐ Refreshed ☐ Somewhat refreshed ☐ Fatigued

Notes
_____
_____
_____

Food Tracking

Breakfast	Servings	Calories	Carbs
Snack			
Lunch			
Snack			
Dinner			
Snack			
TOTAL			

Exercise Tracking

Date _____

	Breakfast		Lunch		Dinner		Bedtime
	Pre	Post	Pre	Post	Pre	Post	
Blood Sugar							
Time							
Insulin Dose							
Medications							

	AM	PM
Blood Pressure		

Sleep Tracking

I went to bed last night at
I got out of bed this morning at
Last night I fell asleep:
　　　☐ Easily　☐ After some time　☐ With difficulty
I woke up during the night:
　　　# of times _____　# of minutes_____
I slept a total of _____ hours
My sleep was disturbed by:

When I woke up for the day, I felt:
　　　☐ Refreshed　☐ Somewhat refreshed　☐ Fatigued

Notes

_____
_____
_____

Food Tracking

Breakfast	Servings	Calories	Carbs
Snack			
Lunch			
Snack			
Dinner			
Snack			
	TOTAL		

Exercise Tracking

Date _____

	Breakfast		Lunch		Dinner		Bedtime
	Pre	Post	Pre	Post	Pre	Post	
Blood Sugar							
Time							
Insulin Dose							
Medications							

	AM	PM
Blood Pressure		

Sleep Tracking

I went to bed last night at
I got out of bed this morning at
Last night I fell asleep:
    ☐ Easily ☐ After some time ☐ With difficulty
I woke up during the night:
    # of times _____ # of minutes_____
I slept a total of _____ hours
My sleep was disturbed by:

When I woke up for the day, I felt:
    ☐ Refreshed ☐ Somewhat refreshed ☐ Fatigued

Notes

_____
_____
_____

Food Tracking

Breakfast	Servings	Calories	Carbs
Snack			
Lunch			
Snack			
Dinner			
Snack			
	TOTAL		

Exercise Tracking

Date _____

| | Breakfast || Lunch || Dinner || Bedtime |
	Pre	Post	Pre	Post	Pre	Post	
Blood Sugar							
Time							
Insulin Dose							
Medications							

	AM	PM
Blood Pressure		

Sleep Tracking

I went to bed last night at
I got out of bed this morning at
Last night I fell asleep:
    ☐ Easily ☐ After some time ☐ With difficulty
I woke up during the night:
    # of times _____ # of minutes_____
I slept a total of _____ hours
My sleep was disturbed by:

When I woke up for the day, I felt:
    ☐ Refreshed ☐ Somewhat refreshed ☐ Fatigued

Notes
_____
_____
_____

Food Tracking

Breakfast	Servings	Calories	Carbs
Snack			
Lunch			
Snack			
Dinner			
Snack			
	TOTAL		

Exercise Tracking

Date _____

| | Breakfast || Lunch || Dinner || Bedtime |
	Pre	Post	Pre	Post	Pre	Post	
Blood Sugar							
Time							
Insulin Dose							
Medications							

	AM	PM
Blood Pressure		

Sleep Tracking

I went to bed last night at
I got out of bed this morning at
Last night I fell asleep:
    ☐ Easily   ☐ After some time   ☐ With difficulty
I woke up during the night:
    # of times _____   # of minutes _____
I slept a total of _____ hours
My sleep was disturbed by:

When I woke up for the day, I felt:
    ☐ Refreshed   ☐ Somewhat refreshed   ☐ Fatigued

Notes

_____
_____
_____

Food Tracking

Breakfast	Servings	Calories	Carbs
Snack			
Lunch			
Snack			
Dinner			
Snack			
TOTAL			

Exercise Tracking

Date _____

| | Breakfast || Lunch || Dinner || Bedtime |
	Pre	Post	Pre	Post	Pre	Post	
Blood Sugar							
Time							
Insulin Dose							
Medications							

	AM	PM
Blood Pressure		

Sleep Tracking

I went to bed last night at
I got out of bed this morning at
Last night I fell asleep:
    ☐ Easily ☐ After some time ☐ With difficulty
I woke up during the night:
    # of times _____ # of minutes_____
I slept a total of _____ hours
My sleep was disturbed by:

When I woke up for the day, I felt:
    ☐ Refreshed ☐ Somewhat refreshed ☐ Fatigued

Notes

_____
_____
_____

Food Tracking

Breakfast	Servings	Calories	Carbs
Snack			
Lunch			
Snack			
Dinner			
Snack			
TOTAL			

Exercise Tracking

Date _____

| | Breakfast || Lunch || Dinner || Bedtime |
	Pre	Post	Pre	Post	Pre	Post	
Blood Sugar							
Time							
Insulin Dose							
Medications							

	AM	PM
Blood Pressure		

Sleep Tracking

I went to bed last night at
I got out of bed this morning at
Last night I fell asleep:
　　　☐ Easily ☐ After some time ☐ With difficulty
I woke up during the night:
　　　# of times _____ # of minutes_____
I slept a total of _____ hours
My sleep was disturbed by:

When I woke up for the day, I felt:
　　　☐ Refreshed ☐ Somewhat refreshed ☐ Fatigued

Notes
_____
_____
_____

Food Tracking

Breakfast	Servings	Calories	Carbs
Snack			
Lunch			
Snack			
Dinner			
Snack			
	TOTAL		

Exercise Tracking

Date _____

| | Breakfast || Lunch || Dinner || Bedtime |
	Pre	Post	Pre	Post	Pre	Post	
Blood Sugar							
Time							
Insulin Dose							
Medications							

	AM	PM
Blood Pressure		

Sleep Tracking

I went to bed last night at
I got out of bed this morning at
Last night I fell asleep:
    ☐ Easily ☐ After some time ☐ With difficulty
I woke up during the night:
    # of times _____ # of minutes_____
I slept a total of _____ hours
My sleep was disturbed by:

When I woke up for the day, I felt:
    ☐ Refreshed ☐ Somewhat refreshed ☐ Fatigued

Notes
_____
_____
_____

Food Tracking

Breakfast	Servings	Calories	Carbs
Snack			
Lunch			
Snack			
Dinner			
Snack			
	TOTAL		

Exercise Tracking

Date _____

	Breakfast		Lunch		Dinner		Bedtime
	Pre	Post	Pre	Post	Pre	Post	
Blood Sugar							
Time							
Insulin Dose							
Medications							

	AM	PM
Blood Pressure		

Sleep Tracking

I went to bed last night at
I got out of bed this morning at
Last night I fell asleep:
    ☐ Easily   ☐ After some time   ☐ With difficulty
I woke up during the night:
    # of times _____   # of minutes _____
I slept a total of _____ hours
My sleep was disturbed by:

When I woke up for the day, I felt:
    ☐ Refreshed   ☐ Somewhat refreshed   ☐ Fatigued

Notes
_____
_____
_____

Food Tracking

Breakfast	Servings	Calories	Carbs
Snack			
Lunch			
Snack			
Dinner			
Snack			
	TOTAL		

Exercise Tracking
_____
_____
_____
_____
_____

Date _____

| | Breakfast || Lunch || Dinner || Bedtime |
	Pre	Post	Pre	Post	Pre	Post	
Blood Sugar							
Time							
Insulin Dose							
Medications							

	AM	PM
Blood Pressure		

Sleep Tracking

I went to bed last night at
I got out of bed this morning at
Last night I fell asleep:
      ☐ Easily ☐ After some time ☐ With difficulty
I woke up during the night:
      # of times _____ # of minutes_____
I slept a total of _____ hours
My sleep was disturbed by:

When I woke up for the day, I felt:
      ☐ Refreshed ☐ Somewhat refreshed ☐ Fatigued

Notes

_____
_____
_____

Food Tracking

Breakfast	Servings	Calories	Carbs
Snack			
Lunch			
Snack			
Dinner			
Snack			
	TOTAL		

Exercise Tracking

Date _____

	Breakfast		Lunch		Dinner		Bedtime
	Pre	Post	Pre	Post	Pre	Post	
Blood Sugar							
Time							
Insulin Dose							
Medications							

	AM	PM
Blood Pressure		

Sleep Tracking

I went to bed last night at
I got out of bed this morning at
Last night I fell asleep:
    ☐ Easily ☐ After some time ☐ With difficulty
I woke up during the night:
    # of times _____ # of minutes_____
I slept a total of _____ hours
My sleep was disturbed by:

When I woke up for the day, I felt:
    ☐ Refreshed ☐ Somewhat refreshed ☐ Fatigued

Notes
_____
_____
_____

Food Tracking

Breakfast	Servings	Calories	Carbs
Snack			
Lunch			
Snack			
Dinner			
Snack			
	TOTAL		

Exercise Tracking

Date _____

| | Breakfast || Lunch || Dinner || Bedtime |
	Pre	Post	Pre	Post	Pre	Post	
Blood Sugar							
Time							
Insulin Dose							
Medications							

	AM	PM
Blood Pressure		

Sleep Tracking

I went to bed last night at
I got out of bed this morning at
Last night I fell asleep:
    ☐ Easily ☐ After some time ☐ With difficulty
I woke up during the night:
    # of times _____   # of minutes_____
I slept a total of _____ hours
My sleep was disturbed by:

When I woke up for the day, I felt:
    ☐ Refreshed ☐ Somewhat refreshed ☐ Fatigued

Notes
_____
_____
_____

Food Tracking

Breakfast	Servings	Calories	Carbs
Snack			
Lunch			
Snack			
Dinner			
Snack			
	TOTAL		

Exercise Tracking

Date _____

| | Breakfast || Lunch || Dinner || Bedtime |
	Pre	Post	Pre	Post	Pre	Post	
Blood Sugar							
Time							
Insulin Dose							
Medications							

	AM	PM
Blood Pressure		

Sleep Tracking

I went to bed last night at
I got out of bed this morning at
Last night I fell asleep:
    ☐ Easily   ☐ After some time   ☐ With difficulty
I woke up during the night:
    # of times _____   # of minutes_____
I slept a total of _____ hours
My sleep was disturbed by:

When I woke up for the day, I felt:
    ☐ Refreshed   ☐ Somewhat refreshed   ☐ Fatigued

Notes
_____
_____
_____

Food Tracking

Breakfast	Servings	Calories	Carbs
Snack			
Lunch			
Snack			
Dinner			
Snack			
TOTAL			

Exercise Tracking

Date _____

| | Breakfast || Lunch || Dinner || Bedtime |
	Pre	Post	Pre	Post	Pre	Post	
Blood Sugar							
Time							
Insulin Dose							
Medications							

	AM	PM
Blood Pressure		

Sleep Tracking

I went to bed last night at
I got out of bed this morning at
Last night I fell asleep:
 ☐ Easily ☐ After some time ☐ With difficulty
I woke up during the night:
 # of times _____ # of minutes_____
I slept a total of _____ hours
My sleep was disturbed by:

When I woke up for the day, I felt:
 ☐ Refreshed ☐ Somewhat refreshed ☐ Fatigued

Notes
_____
_____
_____

Food Tracking

Breakfast	Servings	Calories	Carbs
Snack			
Lunch			
Snack			
Dinner			
Snack			
	TOTAL		

Exercise Tracking

Date _____

	Breakfast		Lunch		Dinner		Bedtime
	Pre	Post	Pre	Post	Pre	Post	
Blood Sugar							
Time							
Insulin Dose							
Medications							

	AM	PM
Blood Pressure		

Sleep Tracking

I went to bed last night at
I got out of bed this morning at
Last night I fell asleep:
    ☐ Easily ☐ After some time ☐ With difficulty
I woke up during the night:
    # of times _____   # of minutes _____
I slept a total of _____ hours
My sleep was disturbed by:

When I woke up for the day, I felt:
    ☐ Refreshed ☐ Somewhat refreshed ☐ Fatigued

Notes
_____
_____
_____

Food Tracking

Breakfast	Servings	Calories	Carbs
Snack			
Lunch			
Snack			
Dinner			
Snack			
	TOTAL		

Exercise Tracking

Date _____

	Breakfast		Lunch		Dinner		Bedtime
	Pre	Post	Pre	Post	Pre	Post	
Blood Sugar							
Time							
Insulin Dose							
Medications							

	AM	PM
Blood Pressure		

Sleep Tracking

I went to bed last night at
I got out of bed this morning at
Last night I fell asleep:
    ☐ Easily ☐ After some time ☐ With difficulty
I woke up during the night:
    # of times _____ # of minutes_____
I slept a total of _____ hours
My sleep was disturbed by:

When I woke up for the day, I felt:
    ☐ Refreshed ☐ Somewhat refreshed ☐ Fatigued

Notes
_____
_____
_____

Food Tracking

Breakfast	Servings	Calories	Carbs
Snack			
Lunch			
Snack			
Dinner			
Snack			
	TOTAL		

Exercise Tracking

Date _____

	Breakfast		Lunch		Dinner		Bedtime
	Pre	Post	Pre	Post	Pre	Post	
Blood Sugar							
Time							
Insulin Dose							
Medications							

	AM	PM
Blood Pressure		

Sleep Tracking

I went to bed last night at
I got out of bed this morning at
Last night I fell asleep:
    ☐ Easily ☐ After some time ☐ With difficulty
I woke up during the night:
    # of times _____ # of minutes_____
I slept a total of _____ hours
My sleep was disturbed by:

When I woke up for the day, I felt:
    ☐ Refreshed ☐ Somewhat refreshed ☐ Fatigued

Notes

_____
_____
_____

Food Tracking

Breakfast	Servings	Calories	Carbs
Snack			
Lunch			
Snack			
Dinner			
Snack			
	TOTAL		

Exercise Tracking

Date _____

| | Breakfast || Lunch || Dinner || Bedtime |
	Pre	Post	Pre	Post	Pre	Post	
Blood Sugar							
Time							
Insulin Dose							
Medications							

	AM	PM
Blood Pressure		

Sleep Tracking

I went to bed last night at
I got out of bed this morning at
Last night I fell asleep:
    ☐ Easily   ☐ After some time   ☐ With difficulty
I woke up during the night:
    # of times _____   # of minutes_____
I slept a total of _____ hours
My sleep was disturbed by:

When I woke up for the day, I felt:
    ☐ Refreshed   ☐ Somewhat refreshed   ☐ Fatigued

Notes

_____
_____
_____

Food Tracking

Breakfast	Servings	Calories	Carbs
Snack			
Lunch			
Snack			
Dinner			
Snack			
TOTAL			

Exercise Tracking

_____
_____
_____
_____
_____

Date _____

	Breakfast		Lunch		Dinner		Bedtime
	Pre	Post	Pre	Post	Pre	Post	
Blood Sugar							
Time							
Insulin Dose							
Medications							

	AM	PM
Blood Pressure		

Sleep Tracking

I went to bed last night at
I got out of bed this morning at
Last night I fell asleep:
    ☐ Easily ☐ After some time ☐ With difficulty
I woke up during the night:
    # of times _____   # of minutes_____
I slept a total of _____ hours
My sleep was disturbed by:

When I woke up for the day, I felt:
    ☐ Refreshed ☐ Somewhat refreshed ☐ Fatigued

Notes
_____
_____
_____

Food Tracking

Breakfast	Servings	Calories	Carbs
Snack			
Lunch			
Snack			
Dinner			
Snack			
	TOTAL		

Exercise Tracking

Date _____

| | Breakfast || Lunch || Dinner || Bedtime |
	Pre	Post	Pre	Post	Pre	Post	
Blood Sugar							
Time							
Insulin Dose							
Medications							

	AM	PM
Blood Pressure		

Sleep Tracking

I went to bed last night at
I got out of bed this morning at
Last night I fell asleep:
    ☐ Easily   ☐ After some time   ☐ With difficulty
I woke up during the night:
    # of times _____   # of minutes_____
I slept a total of _____ hours
My sleep was disturbed by:

When I woke up for the day, I felt:
    ☐ Refreshed   ☐ Somewhat refreshed   ☐ Fatigued

Notes
_____
_____
_____

Food Tracking

Breakfast	Servings	Calories	Carbs
Snack			
Lunch			
Snack			
Dinner			
Snack			
TOTAL			

Exercise Tracking

Date _____

	Breakfast		Lunch		Dinner		Bedtime
	Pre	Post	Pre	Post	Pre	Post	
Blood Sugar							
Time							
Insulin Dose							
Medications							

	AM	PM
Blood Pressure		

Sleep Tracking

I went to bed last night at
I got out of bed this morning at
Last night I fell asleep:
　　　☐ Easily ☐ After some time ☐ With difficulty
I woke up during the night:
　　　# of times _____ # of minutes_____
I slept a total of _____ hours
My sleep was disturbed by:

When I woke up for the day, I felt:
　　　☐ Refreshed ☐ Somewhat refreshed ☐ Fatigued

Notes
_____
_____
_____

Food Tracking

Breakfast	Servings	Calories	Carbs
Snack			
Lunch			
Snack			
Dinner			
Snack			
TOTAL			

Exercise Tracking

Date _____

	Breakfast		Lunch		Dinner		Bedtime
	Pre	Post	Pre	Post	Pre	Post	
Blood Sugar							
Time							
Insulin Dose							
Medications							

	AM	PM
Blood Pressure		

Sleep Tracking

I went to bed last night at
I got out of bed this morning at
Last night I fell asleep:
    ☐ Easily ☐ After some time ☐ With difficulty
I woke up during the night:
    # of times _____ # of minutes_____
I slept a total of _____ hours
My sleep was disturbed by:

When I woke up for the day, I felt:
    ☐ Refreshed ☐ Somewhat refreshed ☐ Fatigued

Notes

_____
_____
_____

Food Tracking

Breakfast	Servings	Calories	Carbs
Snack			
Lunch			
Snack			
Dinner			
Snack			
TOTAL			

Exercise Tracking

_____
_____
_____
_____
_____

Date _____

	Breakfast		Lunch		Dinner		Bedtime
	Pre	Post	Pre	Post	Pre	Post	
Blood Sugar							
Time							
Insulin Dose							
Medications							

	AM	PM
Blood Pressure		

Sleep Tracking

I went to bed last night at
I got out of bed this morning at
Last night I fell asleep:
    ☐ Easily ☐ After some time ☐ With difficulty
I woke up during the night:
    # of times _____ # of minutes_____
I slept a total of _____ hours
My sleep was disturbed by:

When I woke up for the day, I felt:
    ☐ Refreshed ☐ Somewhat refreshed ☐ Fatigued

Notes
_____
_____
_____

Food Tracking

Breakfast	Servings	Calories	Carbs
Snack			
Lunch			
Snack			
Dinner			
Snack			
	TOTAL		

Exercise Tracking

Date _____

	Breakfast		Lunch		Dinner		Bedtime
	Pre	Post	Pre	Post	Pre	Post	
Blood Sugar							
Time							
Insulin Dose							
Medications							

	AM	PM
Blood Pressure		

Sleep Tracking

I went to bed last night at
I got out of bed this morning at
Last night I fell asleep:
☐ Easily ☐ After some time ☐ With difficulty
I woke up during the night:
# of times _____ # of minutes_____
I slept a total of _____ hours
My sleep was disturbed by:

When I woke up for the day, I felt:
☐ Refreshed ☐ Somewhat refreshed ☐ Fatigued

Notes
_____
_____
_____

Food Tracking

Breakfast	Servings	Calories	Carbs
Snack			
Lunch			
Snack			
Dinner			
Snack			
TOTAL			

Exercise Tracking

Date _____

	Breakfast		Lunch		Dinner		Bedtime
	Pre	Post	Pre	Post	Pre	Post	
Blood Sugar							
Time							
Insulin Dose							
Medications							

	AM	PM
Blood Pressure		

Sleep Tracking

I went to bed last night at
I got out of bed this morning at
Last night I fell asleep:
    ☐ Easily   ☐ After some time   ☐ With difficulty
I woke up during the night:
    # of times _____   # of minutes_____
I slept a total of _____ hours
My sleep was disturbed by:

When I woke up for the day, I felt:
    ☐ Refreshed   ☐ Somewhat refreshed   ☐ Fatigued

Notes

_____
_____
_____

Food Tracking

Breakfast	Servings	Calories	Carbs
Snack			
Lunch			
Snack			
Dinner			
Snack			
	TOTAL		

Exercise Tracking

Date _____

	Breakfast		Lunch		Dinner		Bedtime
	Pre	Post	Pre	Post	Pre	Post	
Blood Sugar							
Time							
Insulin Dose							
Medications							

	AM	PM
Blood Pressure		

Sleep Tracking

I went to bed last night at
I got out of bed this morning at
Last night I fell asleep:
    ☐ Easily ☐ After some time ☐ With difficulty
I woke up during the night:
    # of times _____ # of minutes_____
I slept a total of _____ hours
My sleep was disturbed by:

When I woke up for the day, I felt:
    ☐ Refreshed ☐ Somewhat refreshed ☐ Fatigued

Notes
_____
_____
_____

Food Tracking

Breakfast	Servings	Calories	Carbs
Snack			
Lunch			
Snack			
Dinner			
Snack			
	TOTAL		

Exercise Tracking

Date _____

| | Breakfast || Lunch || Dinner || Bedtime |
	Pre	Post	Pre	Post	Pre	Post	
Blood Sugar							
Time							
Insulin Dose							
Medications							

	AM	PM
Blood Pressure		

Sleep Tracking

I went to bed last night at
I got out of bed this morning at
Last night I fell asleep:
    ☐ Easily ☐ After some time ☐ With difficulty
I woke up during the night:
    # of times _____ # of minutes_____
I slept a total of _____ hours
My sleep was disturbed by:

When I woke up for the day, I felt:
    ☐ Refreshed ☐ Somewhat refreshed ☐ Fatigued

Notes
_____
_____
_____

Food Tracking

Breakfast	Servings	Calories	Carbs
Snack			
Lunch			
Snack			
Dinner			
Snack			
	TOTAL		

Exercise Tracking

Date _____

	Breakfast		Lunch		Dinner		Bedtime
	Pre	Post	Pre	Post	Pre	Post	
Blood Sugar							
Time							
Insulin Dose							
Medications							

	AM	PM
Blood Pressure		

Sleep Tracking

I went to bed last night at
I got out of bed this morning at
Last night I fell asleep:
 ☐ Easily ☐ After some time ☐ With difficulty
I woke up during the night:
 # of times _____ # of minutes _____
I slept a total of _____ hours
My sleep was disturbed by:

When I woke up for the day, I felt:
 ☐ Refreshed ☐ Somewhat refreshed ☐ Fatigued

Notes

_____
_____
_____

Food Tracking

Breakfast	Servings	Calories	Carbs
Snack			
Lunch			
Snack			
Dinner			
Snack			
	TOTAL		

Exercise Tracking

Date _____

	Breakfast		Lunch		Dinner		Bedtime
	Pre	Post	Pre	Post	Pre	Post	
Blood Sugar							
Time							
Insulin Dose							
Medications							

	AM	PM
Blood Pressure		

Sleep Tracking

I went to bed last night at
I got out of bed this morning at
Last night I fell asleep:
 ☐ Easily ☐ After some time ☐ With difficulty
I woke up during the night:
 # of times _____   # of minutes_____
I slept a total of _____ hours
My sleep was disturbed by:

When I woke up for the day, I felt:
 ☐ Refreshed ☐ Somewhat refreshed ☐ Fatigued

Notes
_____
_____
_____

Food Tracking

Breakfast	Servings	Calories	Carbs
Snack			
Lunch			
Snack			
Dinner			
Snack			
TOTAL			

Exercise Tracking

Blood Pressure Tracker

Date	AM	PM

Date	AM	PM

Date	AM	PM

Date	AM	PM

Thanks

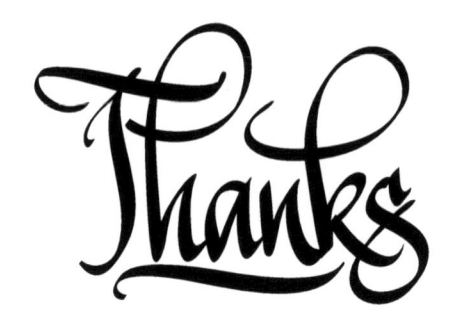

We hope you found this log book useful.
For more log books, journals, and planners by **Bold Visions**,
please visit https://amzn.to/32W1v7D..

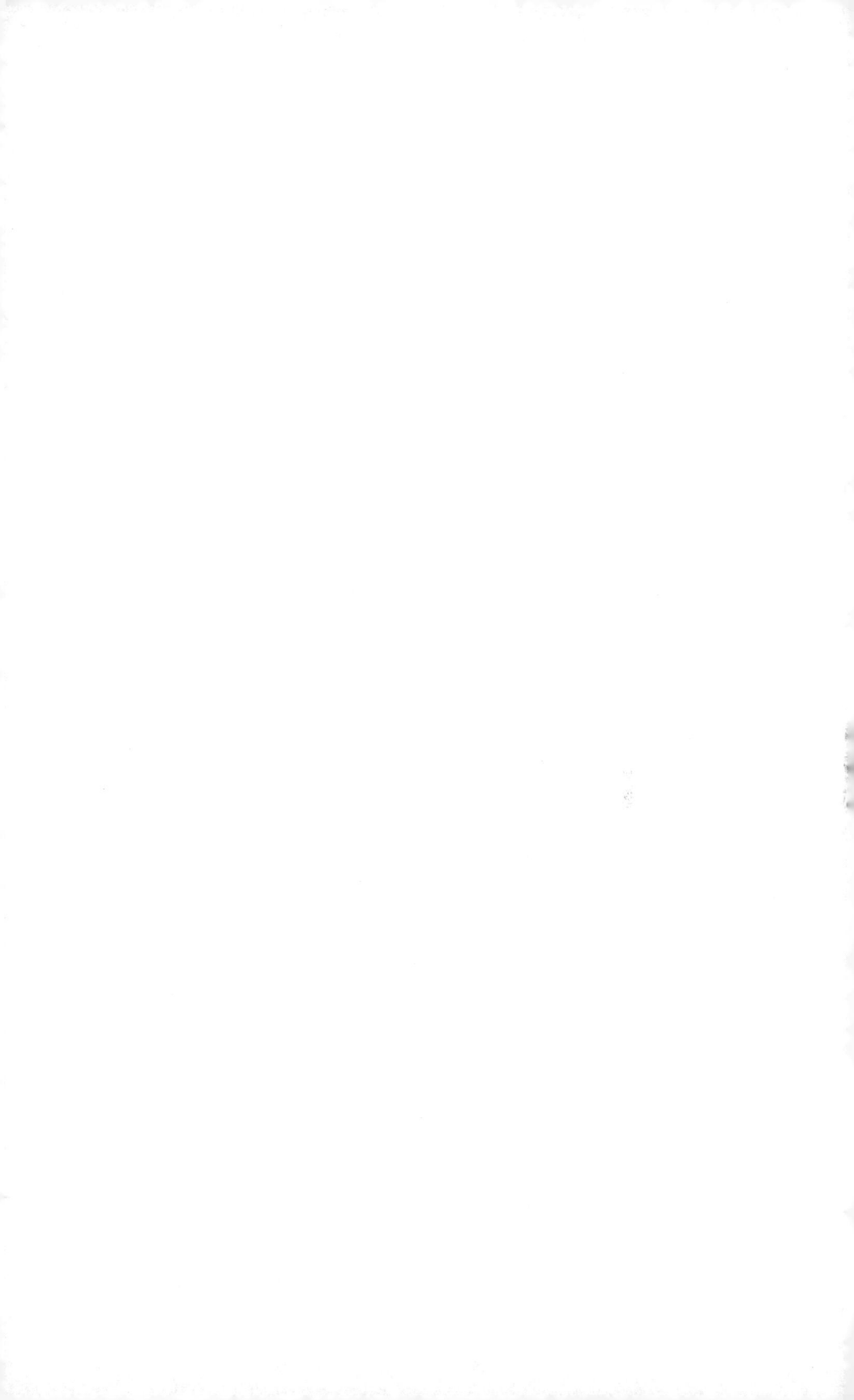

Made in the USA
Columbia, SC
27 July 2022